MR. JONES' AUTOGRAPH

If it appears here, someone loves and respects you a great deal. Mr. Jones is very shy and reclusive; his autograph is almost impossible to obtain!

D1503091

MEDICARE

FOR THE LAZY MAN

2023

SIMPLEST & EASIEST GUIDE EVER!

DOUGLAS B. JONES
CLU, RHU

MEDICARE
FOR THE LAZY MAN

SIMPLEST & EASIEST GUIDE EVER!

2023

WHAT READERS SAY:

Simple. Straightforward. Funny. The Only Book to Buy About Medicare.
> — TexasCyclistg

...do not miss reading this book... it's pretty much all you need to know.
> — Hummingbyrd

...he's one of the few out there who is protecting your interest. Truly.
> — Clemuel

I bought this book for the cover. Little did I know how practical and applicable it is.
> — Vincente C. Santiago

Makes signing up for Medicare almost fun! I love Douglas' brevity and humor.
> — Gyroqueen

The best and most transparent source of information on Medicare I have come across.
> — Doug V. Jr.

Easy to understand and Doug personally answered the specific questions I had!

— John M.

IT DELIVERS... A MONEY SAVER, GREAT BOOK.

— Michael S.

Great guide to getting good Medicare coverage.

— Tim McCarthy

Great book, great author...

— Jude

I would also highly recommend Doug's podcasts; they are both entertaining and informative.

— Dominick Regina

It's clever, insightful, and is helpful in overcoming "Medicare Anxiety."

— Svea Darnall

...the recommendations are simply brilliant.

— Don Pisto

THIS BOOK IS DEDICATED TO:
LAZY MEN and LAZY LADIES, too smart to
waste time and energy on stupidity!

It was written expressly for Medicare eligible Americans who:

- Are not infirm, but want to ensure that protections are in place if infirmity strikes.

- Are not destitute but intend to get maximum value from the money spent on Medicare coverages.

- Want to understand cost-effective ways to defend against catastrophic financial impact of medical treatment.

- Most of all, seek a simple and clear explanation of Medicare in order to make the best possible choices.

Is it time to buy Medicare insurance?

Would you like me to assist you?

Go to:

WWW.MEDICAREFORTHELAZYMAN.COM

Securely complete & send me short questionnaire.

(Or email: DBJ@MLMMailbag.com)

There is never a charge for my professional advice.

Try out my podcast:

Medicare for the Lazy Man Podcast

Wherever fine podcasts are given away free of charge!

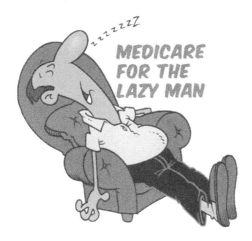

CONTENTS

INTRODUCTION 1

CHAPTER 1: Do Normal People Really Read This Stuff? 7

CHAPTER 2: What the Heck Does Medicare Do? 10

CHAPTER 3: Introducing: Your Insurance Agent 13

CHAPTER 4: Medicare Part A 17

CHAPTER 5: Medicare Part B 19

CHAPTER 6: Sources of Information 23

CHAPTER 7: Medicare is Not Enough Protection! 26

CHAPTER 8: Medicare Supplement Plans 29

CHAPTER 9: The Best Kept Secret in Medicare 35

CHAPTER 10: Medicare Advantage (Part C) Plans 38

CHAPTER 11: Medicare MSA 42

CHAPTER 12: Drugs? We Don't Need No Stinkin' Drugs! 45

CHAPTER 13: What Will All of This Cost? 50

CHAPTER 14: Massachusetts, Minnesota & Wisconsin 53

CHAPTER 15: The Only Chapter You Are Likely to Need! 58

CHAPTER 16: Did You Make a Boo-Boo? 64

ACKNOWLEDGMENTS 66

ABOUT THE AUTHOR 68

INTRODUCTION

Welcome to the 2023 version of Medicare for the Lazy Man! This is the sixth edition of a work that strives to make the reader's transition to Medicare a more pleasant one.

This massive Federal program was created back in the 1960s with the aim of helping older Americans cope with the rapidly rising cost of health insurance. A noble goal, but over the decades it has blown up into a complex and often confusing bureaucracy that can be frustrating to its intended beneficiaries.

Why does Medicare operate in a seemingly nonsensical way?

- Some genius decided Medicare should imitate the very first health insurance plans ever created, back in the mist-shrouded dawn of history.

- The program has always been a political football.

- Government functionaries reject the superior examples set by private industry; insurance companies have the expertise and motivation to perform the same functions better, cheaper and much more cheerfully.

So, the government created its own insurance company. In the process it also laid the foundation for a pervasive myth that is subscribed to by many of the people approaching Medicare age.

The myth in question holds that:

1. Unless one learns about every little aspect of the program there is a risk of errors.

2. These errors will cause disaster and doom that will haunt one for the rest of one's miserable, wretched life.

I am here to reassure you that this is not true. There is no reason to fear the arrival of Medicare; it is likely to be a very positive change in your life.

In the Obamacare world of health insurance for those who are pre-Medicare, the available protection is often skimpy and very expensive.

When I first learned about group medical insurance, a monthly premium of around $10 would buy coverage for a 30-39 year-old with a $500 deductible, an unlimited lifetime maximum and with no restrictive provider network of doctors and hospitals.

That kind of value is a thing of the past everywhere except under Medicare. Fortunately, politicians who caused disaster in the health insurance markets did not have the political courage to destroy this program that continues to provide a good benefit for the price its participants are charged.

So long as Medicare remains a political "third rail", those who enter its portals will discover that much of what they find in Medicare Land will be cause for celebration!

Those celebrants, by the way, comprise a very large and growing tribe. We Baby Boomers (born 1946 to 1964) are a population cohort that looks like a fat rat passing through a snake. There is a great deal of money to be earned by selling us insurance to protect against the gaps in Medicare coverage.

Normal people view Medicare as an impenetrable mass of complexities. Most who are approaching age 65 would very much like to avoid having to study and learn about health insurance but fear that would result in poor choices and a lifetime of misery.

There is one class of abnormal people who purport to have studied and memorized mountains of Medicare minutia. They expect to be referred to as "consultants", "advisors" and "experts". Of course they do!

In my view, many of them are just "leeches". They routinely troll for fresh victims who will buy their commission-rich Medicare Advantage products. The leeches will razzle-dazzle their targets with snake-oil salesmanship, resulting in an aging population that is burdened with inferior protection.

These people are licensed agents and we are forced to purchase from them because the states have mandated it so. The commissions to be earned from selling us Medicare-related insurance represent a substantial source of income for the insurance agent.

By now you may have realized that I am also a leech, an agent licensed in all 50 states. I love to earn commission dollars and view my fellow Boomers with much fiscal lust in my heart. However, the advice offered to my clients and readers has some major differences from what they are likely to receive from my fellow leeches.

My advice:

1. is much shorter and easier to grasp

2. may offer a bigger bang from the bucks you spend.

3. allows you to tell an agent exactly what you intend to purchase (and why).

Studying all of the minutia about Medicare is likely to be a huge waste of time and effort... unless you enjoy that sort of thing, of course.

Why? Because knowledge does NOT equal power! Nothing you memorize about Medicare will allow you to improve it in order to get better or cheaper protection. Also, any implication that disaster will ensue if your Medicare choices are not absolutely perfect is equally false.

In reality, very few Medicare decisions are completely irrevocable; mistakes and poor choices can often be fixed within a year or less.

Generally, the costliest mistakes actually stem from refusal to act, as in the case of late enrollment penalties. Later on, I provide a step-by-step guide to Medicare enrollment and the acquisition of related insurance that will complete the process for the majority of readers in average circumstances.

Look for "**The only chapter you are likely to need**" near the end of this book for a synopsis of my recommendations.

NOMENCLATURE: PARTS vs. PLANS

Original Medicare consisted of two elements called PARTS

PART A – covers **inpatient** treatment in a hospital or skilled nursing facility, hospice and home health care

PART B – covers **outpatient** treatment in doctors' offices, diagnostic testing, emergency treatment, etc.

Added to the Medicare program more recently are:

PART C – So called "Medicare Advantage" plans (MA & MAPD) which I do not recommend

PART D – Prescription Drug Plans (PDP) defray some of the cost of prescription medications

Coverages that supplement Medicare are called PLANS:

MEDICARE SUPPLEMENT PLANS – protect against the gaps in Medicare

PRESCRIPTION DRUG PLANS – PDPs which defray some of the cost of prescription medications

IN THIS BOOK I ONLY RECOMMEND:

MEDICARE PART A

MEDICARE PART B

MEDICARE SUPPLEMENT PLANS

PRESCRIPTION DRUG PLANS

These four provide the best protection available.

CHAPTER 1

Do normal people really read this stuff?

Why have you decided to buy (or shoplift) this book?

- Are you closing in on Medicare age?
- Leaving job-related group insurance?
- Responsible for advising a friend or relative?
- Reexamining choices you made in the past?
- Suffering from insomnia?
- Paying the price for a dissolute life?

Are you seeking a quick roadmap through the Medicare maze?

What is your destination?

Until I dragged her out west to the University of Arizona, my wife attended a Catholic grade school and Jr. High, a Catholic girl's academy and a Catholic women's college.

Eventually I realized that Catholic schools do not teach geography because she cannot navigate her way out of a wet paper bag.

However, if you treat this book like a map and follow my suggestions, you will be able to easily navigate to your goal of selecting and acquiring the essential layers of coverage necessary for protection under Medicare:

MEDICARE PART A

MEDICARE PART B

MEDICARE SUPPLEMENT PLANS

PRESCRIPTION DRUG PLANS

That is all you need for complete protection, and it is very likely that these coverages will serve you well for the many decades of life you have yet to enjoy.

There will be no need to do an annual review or renewal for anything except perhaps the Prescription Drug Plan (PDP) and then only if you want to make sure yours is the least costly plan available.

Aiming to simplify a complex subject.

If that simplification is successful it should relieve the angst many feel when the time comes to make decisions about Medicare coverage.

Generally, there are three groups of people that may benefit most by considering the recommendations they will find here:

1. Those aged 64 who are preparing for initial Medicare enrollment.

2. Those aged 65 or older who are planning to leave their current employer sponsored insurance plan.

3. Existing Medicare participants who want to consider improving the quality or cost of their coverage.

Within these pages the average citizen confronting Medicare for the first time will discover a short, direct path from start to finish that will relieve their concerns and likely save some money.

Notice I said "average citizen". The recommendations in this book are not for everyone, but the vast majority of those approaching

Medicare eligibility will be well served by these suggestions.

My book has been written for those with:

Average or better health

Average or better financial resources

No desire to waste time or effort studying Medicare

Most helped will be people responsible for their own health insurance, specifically those about to turn 65 and employed people 65+ contemplating retirement or termination from an employer's health insurance plan.

Those who are stricken with debilitating medical conditions generally have an active support system to assist them in making Medicare decisions. In my lengthy experience, very few people with disabilities have asked me for assistance, leading me to believe that they are well served by local experts who are tasked with providing guidance. Make no mistake, the advice offered in this book leads to the finest Medicare coverages available on the market today so all readers will benefit, no matter their state of health.

People who are in dire financial straits should drop this book immediately and seek advice from their state's Medicaid (welfare) office. Though funded largely by the Federal government, the Medicaid program is administered by the states so the qualifications and requirements differ widely from one jurisdiction to another.

Once again, if you are destitute, stop reading right now and try to get a refund. This book is not for you!

CHAPTER 2

WHAT THE HECK DOES MEDICARE DO?

If you spent some of the 1960s within range of WLS-AM 890, Chicago's 50,000-watt rock blowtorch, you probably heard the legend of a very lazy young guy named Hootie Sapperticker. DJ Art Roberts promoted June 22 as Hootie Sapperticker Day, but the campaign never really gained traction and Hootie eventually faded into obscurity.

Decades later, Hootie and the Mrs. turned age 65 and, with my guidance, signed up for Medicare through the government on its "oh so user-friendly" website.

Because they learned that Medicare coverage is full of gaps and cost sharing, they also purchased insurance to protect themselves from those weaknesses in the program - insurance to supplement Medicare known as a Medicare supplement. Clever, huh?

As luck would have it, Mr. & Mrs. Sapperticker have a cute little grandchild who spends part of every day in a bubbling germ factory called nursery school. After enjoying hugs and kisses from this grandchild, they each contracted a major dose of the most virulent flu of the season. Surviving this disease required visits to a hospital ER, laboratory testing and several follow-up appointments with the family doctor after being released from confinement.

Hooty Sapperticker expected massive medical bills to start arriving shortly after treatment, but that did not happen. Because they are protected by Medicare, the invoices from the hospital, the doctors, the laboratory etc. were all sent to the federal government for payment. That process started as the patients showed their ID cards to office staff when treatment began.

After calculating and paying their share, the government

functionaries (in the guise of Medicare) sent notification to the insurance company that issued their Medicare Supplement policies. The clerks at the insurance company double-checked the government calculations and then issued payment to the providers of medical treatment for the balances due them.

Months after their full recovery, the financial consequences of their illness were resolved. The very conservative Mrs. Sapperticker had purchased the Cadillac of Medicare supplement plans and paid a monthly premium of around $150. She was delighted to find that her medical bills were paid in full except for a small annual deductible of $226 – almost 100% coverage.

On the other hand, Hooty has always been more of a risk-taking party animal. He had purchased the High-Deductible Plan G (HDG) Medicare supplement plan for about $35 per month.

Hooty had to write checks for a few hundred dollars in cost sharing because of the very reasonable deductible his plan carries, but this was more than offset by the $100+ he saves each month in lower premiums. In addition, his beer funds have been protected from bill collectors.

The happy conclusion is that I, as the Sapperticker family insurance advisor, have been elevated to heroic status and toasted in absentia every time they gather together.

The cute little grandchild was never told about all of the misery caused by his grandparents' unconditional love.

SO, WHAT IS THE BIG DEAL ABOUT MEDICARE, ANYWAY?

Now that we understand Medicare is a simple bill paying mechanism for those Americans it covers, why is there such a hoo-rah about it?

Hapless citizens in their middle sixties are accosted with piles of insurance company propaganda and endless telephone calls warning about the dangers of charging into Medicare without their professional guidance. Washed-up celebrities add to the confusion by exhorting viewers to dial a toll-free number to "get what you deserve". Lengthy lists of "free benefits" are recited in these advertisements, the implication being that they might have become available in the viewer's area.

I have spoken to some who were victimized by these unscrupulous charlatans and the negative results were two-fold. The hard-sell tactics were almost brutal and the products being pushed are designed to pay the largest sales commission rather than to accommodate the buyer's needs. My view of the evolving sales tactics in this field of insurance is that altruism is a rare commodity and the most successful agents work on volume, volume, volume!

It is really all about the commissions, folks!

This is why you will be buried in pitches for Medicare Advantage plans that have the richest commissions, followed by much smaller piles of come-ons for Medicare Supplement plans that have less generous commission schedules by which insurance agents are paid.

However, you will never be told about my favorite plan, the best kept secret in all of Medicare. In order to force a discussion about the plan I most often recommend, you will have to grab the typical agent by the lapels and say the magic words: **high deductible**.

More about this closely guarded secret later in the book.

CHAPTER 3

INTRODUCING:
YOUR INSURANCE AGENT

Way back in the last millennium I joined the family business, and passed the Illinois insurance license examination. The large room was full of test-takers and I would like to think a majority of them passed with the minimum score of 70%. What happened next?

Well, some went on to a life of admirable servitude to hordes of grateful clients and then spent a prosperous retirement enjoying the fruits of their success. Others found non-sales positions within the ranks of insurance company clerical staff, from which a few executives are eventually plucked. The rest were thrown to the wolves and landed on the heap of insurance company casualties in fairly short order. Eventually they moved on to other fields of endeavor.

Meanwhile, the insurance machine continues devouring masses of humanity, attempting to turn them into super-salesmen. This is a universal quest and one of the great mysteries of insurance: how can we identify, recruit and motivate candidates who are most likely to succeed in this cutthroat business?

There are many desperate insurance agents out there who have fallen victim to empty promises of easy success and these people will do just about anything to make a sale and earn a few dollars. Desperate people sometimes do desperate things.

Scattered through this book I express several related thoughts:

- **Medicare supplement** plans provide superior protection against financial loss from unexpected medical expenses.

- Agents are paid a higher commission when the product you

purchase, like **Plan G**, is more expensive.

- The inexpensive **High Deductible Plan G (HDG)** is the best, most cost-effective Medicare supplement plan for almost everyone.

- You are unlikely to ever be told about the **High Deductible** option because most agents intend to maximize their income by selling **Plan G** exclusively.

If you agree with my statements (above), the inescapable conclusion is that most people looking for the best Medicare guidance are being ill-served by desperate agents. However, those insurance applications have to be signed by licensed agents, according to state law, so let's look at the way we would like YOUR agent to operate.

1. Early in the relationship, your agent should learn about you, your current situation, your desires and expectations for Medicare coverage.

2. Your agent should illustrate the cost of insurance products that will best meet your needs and satisfy your expectations.

3. The insurance companies selected to offer the products should be fiscally sound and responsible, providing responsive customer service when needed.

4. When you have enough information to make confident decisions, your agent should make the application process as easy for you as possible.

5. After the underwriting and approval steps have been completed, your agent should notify you of this and the impending arrival of policy documents with ID cards.

6. Your agent now has an ongoing obligation. He must make himself available to answer questions and provide advice and service anytime this might be helpful to you, his valued client.

Doug Jones, your new agent?
ABSOLUTELY NO CHARGE TO YOU!

Medicare will not allow me to handle your Parts A & B enrollment, but you should have no problem if you follow the instructions in the relevant chapters. If I am lucky enough to be asked to serve as your insurance agent, I will make it easy and painless to acquire the other essential layers of insurance protection. You may contact me here:

www.MedicareForTheLazyMan.com

DBJ@MedicareForTheLazyMan.com

On the landing page of my website you will find a yellow button shouting: "Get A Quote". Click that button to find a short questionnaire that asks a few demographic facts about you. When you have answered the questions and entered any additional comments you want to share, click the "submit" button and the form will be sent directly to me in a very secure manner.

Or send an e-mail with any comments or requests you care to share with me. You probably aren't an insurance expert so you may overlook some necessary details. Likely I will send you a short questionnaire asking for supporting information, which will allow me to accurately quote the cost of Medicare supplement insurance.

I may also send a questionnaire requesting detail on your prescription medications and preferred pharmacies. Once I have that information, I can use the government database to identify the least expensive Prescription Drug Plan (PDP) available in your area. If you like, perform the same search yourself using the steps outlined elsewhere in this book.

When discussing insurance products, I will probably send you legally required documents such as brochures, Outlines of Coverage and government pamphlets.

Once you and I agree on the products you wish to purchase, I will send you a simple questionnaire that, when completed and returned to me, will supply the information I need to fill out the otherwise confusing insurance applications. When combined with the signature pages you will execute, I will securely fax the applications to the insurance company(s) and send complete copies to you.

This painless process will be over shortly and you will have acquired the finest health insurance available in the Medicare marketplace today!

CHAPTER 4

Medicare Part A

Your goal in buying, borrowing or stealing this book should be to minimize the time and effort required to select and establish your Medicare related coverages. Let's get after it!

MEDICARE PART A is health insurance provided by the Federal government. It is intended to reimburse most of the expenses incurred during treatment in an inpatient facility (hospital, skilled nursing and rehabilitation) as well as hospice and limited home health care.

In almost all cases, Americans with a 10-year work history (or those married to someone with a 10-year history of taxable employment) will have Part A provided to them free of charge.

Since it is free, almost everyone is advised to enroll in Part A coincident with their 65th birth month (note the HSA exception below). That coverage effective date (as with all Medicare-related coverages) will be on the first of the month in question.

Generally, someone approaching age 65 may enroll up to three months before the birthday month begins. Coverage will then go into effect on the 1st day of that birth month. Since Part A is almost always free of charge, completing the enrollment as early as possible is the most prudent choice.

One also has three months available to enroll after the birth month, but this could mean going without coverage for a period. It also means that some Federal bureaucrat will select the Part A start date according to incomprehensible rules only he has access to. If disenrollment from an employer's group insurance plan is contemplated, it is best to check with SSA to ensure that Medicare's start will be coordinated with your current plan's end.

Exception: if the actual date of birth is on the 1st of any month, eligibility for coverage is moved forward one month and the Medicare participant will become effective on the 1st day of the prior month.

Don't ask why this is so; nobody knows.

Exception: if the existing health insurance plan is an HSA (Health Savings Account) and you intend to continue making tax advantaged contributions, regulations prohibit enrollment in any part of Medicare during that period.

ENROLL IN MEDICARE PART A ONLINE HERE:
https://www.ssa.gov/medicare/

(SSA is the Social Security Administration, the government agency originally charged with overseeing the Medicare program.)

Scroll down to the blue button: Apply for Medicare Only

How To Apply Online for Just Medicare

If you are within three months of age 65 or older and not ready to start your monthly Social Security benefits yet, you can use our online retirement application to sign up just for Medicare and wait to apply for your retirement or spouses benefits later. It takes less than 10 minutes, and there are no forms to sign and usually no documentation is required.

Apply for Medicare Only

Return to Saved Application | Check Application

Status | Replace Medicare Card

To find out what documents and information you need to apply, go to the Checklist For The Online Medicare, Retirement, and Spouses Application.

CHAPTER 5

Medicare Part B

At the risk of belaboring the obvious, the following is my official definition of the second part of Medicare:

MEDICARE PART B is health insurance provided by the Federal government. It is generally intended to reimburse expenses incurred during treatment by doctors, typically in an outpatient setting, as well as testing & diagnostics, medical equipment, supplies and preventive care.

It is important to choose the effective date of your Part B coverage very carefully. Medicare Part B carries a substantial monthly premium (starting at $164.90/month in 2023) so it would not be prudent to start it too early.

More important, since Medicare Part B is critically important protection designed to reimburse the costs of the most commonly encountered treatment, it would REALLY not be prudent to enroll too late.

Late enrollment in Part B, after becoming eligible, risks incurring hefty medical expenses without insurance protection. If one fails to enroll until after the eligibility period, the opportunity to enroll may be limited. In addition, substantially late enrollment in Part B subjects one to a lifetime monetary penalty that will be added to the monthly premium forever.

The importance of timely Part B enrollment cannot be stated too strongly.

Turning age 65:

Medicare eligible people who are responsible for their own health insurance will have no difficulty choosing an enrollment date. They will turn age 65 and will properly enroll with an effective date of the first day of their 65th birth month.

Exception: if the actual date of birth is on the 1st of any month, coverage will become effective on the 1st day of the prior month.

Don't ask why this is so; nobody knows.

The enrollment period begins 3 months before the birth month, and prudence dictates that the enrollment process should begin as early as practical within that 90-day period.

Exception: Employed people (and their spouses) who are covered by an employer sponsored group insurance plan that is considered "creditable" need not worry about Medicare enrollment when turning 65 until they are preparing to retire or disenroll from that plan. At this time, they will have a special enrollment period (SEP) which will allow them to enroll in Medicare without concern about health history or late enrollment penalty.

Retirement or departure from an employer's group medical plan after turning 65:

Medicare coverages should be scheduled to begin when the group plan terminates. It is not prudent to have any gap in coverage and it is really bad to have a gap lasting longer than 63 continuous days. At that point your medical history might come into play as to when you will be allowed to have full coverage for pre-existing medical conditions.

Neither insurance coverage under COBRA nor retiree health insurance offered by your employer qualifies as a substitute for Part B enrollment.

The enrollment application used for Medicare Part B is: CMS-40B and may be downloaded from numerous locations, including MedicareForTheLazyMan.com. It will be important to confirm that there was health insurance coverage in place just prior to the requested Part B effectivedate.

The form used to verify prior coverage is CMS – L564. It may be downloaded from numerous locations in the internet, including MedicareForTheLazyMan.com.

During the current virus panic some enrollment rules have been liberalized so the employer's signature on the CMS-L564 is not currently required.

Other circumstances that might affect your coverage decisions:

- Do you have a spouse who is actively employed?

- Are you not a US citizen?

- Are you on COBRA or retiree medical coverage from an employer group plan?

- Are you eligible for Tricare or other VA coverage?

- Do you fall into another category that complicates things?

If any of the above apply, you may need professional advice about whether, or exactly when to begin Medicare Part B coverage. I am always happy to offer assistance, plus you might find reliable advice in the list of resources in the following chapter.

ENROLL IN MEDICARE PART B ONLINE HERE:

https://www.ssa.gov/medicare/

(SSA is the Social Security Administration, the government agency originally charged with overseeing the Medicare program. They use the word "retirement" repeatedly to mean Social Security.)

Scroll down to this section just above the blue "Apply" button:

Should I Sign Up For Medical Insurance (Part B)?

With our online application, you can sign up for Medicare Part A (hospital insurance) and Part B (medical insurance). Because you must pay a premium for Part B coverage, you can turn it down.

If you're eligible at age 65, your initial enrollment period begins three months before your 65th birthday, includes the month you turn age 65, and ends three months after that birthday.

If you choose not to enroll in Medicare Part B and then decide to do so later, your coverage could be delayed and you may have to pay a higher monthly premium for as long as you have Part B. Your monthly premium will go up 10 percent for each 12-month period you were eligible for Part B, but didn't sign up for it, unless you qualify for a "Special Enrollment Period" (SEP).

If you don't enroll in Medicare Part B during your initial enrollment period, you have another chance each year to sign up during a "general enrollment period" from January 1 through March 31. Your coverage begins on July 1 of the year you enroll. Read our Medicare publication for more information.

If you have a Health Savings Account (HSA) or health insurance based on current employment, you may want to ask your personnel office or insurance company how signing up for Medicare will affect you.

If the online enrollment becomes problematic, I suggest calling the nearest office of the Social Security Administration to ask how they suggest you proceed with the enrollment process and the submission of the required documents.

It appears to me that there is a lack of consistency in how enrollments are being facilitated presently, so it is best to ask for instructions from those who will be in charge of the procedures.

CHAPTER 6

SOURCES OF INFORMATION

Here are some (theoretically) unbiased sources of information and advice on choosing the proper Medicare effective date for you/your spouse:

Choosing a Medigap Policy: A Guide to Health Insurance for People with Medicare:

https://www.medicare.gov/media/9486

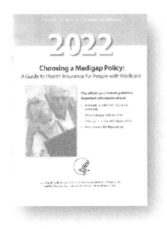

Helpful contacts in each state www.Medicare.gov/contacts

SSA: The Social Security Administration (which administers the Medicare program)

https://www.ssa.gov/medicare/

Enrolling in Medicare Part A & Part B

www.medicare.gov/Pubs/pdf/11036-Enrolling-Medicare-Part-A-Part-B.pdf

CMS Product No. 11036

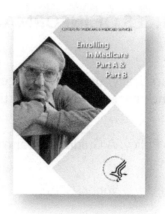

Medicare & You 2023:

www.medicare.gov/Pubs/pdf/10050-medicare-and-you.pdf

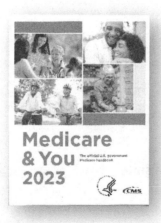

Medicare for Dummies Cheat Sheet

https://www.dummies.com/article/business-careers-money/personal-finance/medicare/medicare-for-dummies-cheat-sheet-207834

SHIP – State Health Insurance Assistance Programs – choose your state from the drop-down menu

https://www.shiptacenter.org/

Public service agencies, like a local hospital for instance, may have a Medicare and Social Security advisor on staff.

Your company HR department

CHAPTER 7

Medicare Is Not Enough Protection!

If you have started the Medicare enrollment process with plenty of time to spare before the effective or starting date, of your coverage, take a break. Do something more fun or productive until confirmation of your successful enrollment arrives.

This confirmation could be in the form of a Medicare ID card received in the US mail, or even sooner, a "Benefit Verification Letter" deposited without warning in your online, password protected account that they asked you to set up.

It will show your unique alpha/numeric "identifier" and the start dates for Parts A and B. Each will provide confirmation of your participation in Medicare should you ever need to prove it to a medical provider's staff.

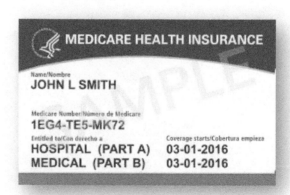

Now is the time to purchase the insurance that will protect you from the dangerous gaping holes in Medicare coverage.

What are these gaping holes you ask? They are the deductibles, coinsurance, and unlimited lifetime cost sharing amounts that severely limit the protection afforded by original Medicare.

These cost sharing elements of Medicare Part A and Part B have no statutory limit. Potentially, very large amounts of money are at risk for people on Medicare who have not purchased additional protection from a private insurance company. Someone once calculated that, if everything that could go wrong did go wrong over $900,000 in medical expenses could be charged to a Medicare participant who was only covered by original Medicare.

Insurance to supplement Medicare

Two basic types of insurance are available to protect you from financial disaster. One is clearly superior.

1. **MEDICARE SUPPLEMENT PLANS** – The best and only choice for health insurance to supplement Medicare, assuming you can afford a modest monthly premium cost.

Medicare supplement plans range from very comprehensive to very cost effective. In keeping with my goal of simplification, I have only recommended the very richest Plan G or the streamlined High Deductible Plan G (HDG). People who turned 65 before 2020 (born before 1955) may select HDF instead of HDG, but the insurance companies seem to be ratcheting up the premiums on their regular Plans F so those are rapidly losing their allure.

If you are a youngster who first turned 65 in 2020 or later, the simplest and most comprehensive supplement plan available to you will be Plan G. The most cost-effective plan you will be allowed to purchase will be the brand-new High Deductible Plan G (HDG). These two plans operate just like their predecessors (F and HDF) except that Plan G does not cover the Part B annual deductible, which is $226 during the year 2023.

MEDICARE SUPPLEMENTS GIVE YOU FREEDOM!

Read the next two chapters (8 & 9) to learn why I only recommend Medicare supplements to all of my clients.

2. **MEDICARE ADVANTAGE PLANS (PART C)** – Do not even consider these or waste your time learning about them.

This type of supplemental coverage actually removes Medicare Parts A & B, along with their benefits and protections. Original Medicare is replaced by an insurance company plan that forces participants into an HMO-like gulag of rules, regulations and restrictions. The only reason you hear about Medicare Advantage plans so often is that they pay very generous commissions to the insurance agent thanks in large part to you, the American taxpayer.

You can read more about Medicare Advantage (Part C) in Chapter 10 if you have some time to kill.

CHAPTER 8

Medicare Supplement Plans:

The ONLY Way to Fly!

When compared with the highly-flawed Medicare Advantage (Part C) plans, Medicare supplement plans have only one disadvantage: they are not given away free of charge.

Each Medicare supplement plan has a monthly premium charge, although the costs vary widely between states, insurance carriers and type of plan.

The available plans are standardized from company to company and state to state. Each is denoted by a letter, so as an example, Plan A provides the same protections and benefits no matter which company sells it and no matter which state it is sold in.

In almost all states there are as many as twelve Medicare Supplement plans being sold, and they all have one great thing in common:

COMPLETE FREEDOM OF CHOICE!

1. Medicare supplement plans never have restrictive networks of doctors and hospitals.

    A person covered by a Medicare supplement plan is free to seek treatment from any provider anywhere (in the USA or possessions) who accepts Medicare patients. The greatest medical specialists in the world practice in various facilities around the United States and none of them have been placed out of reach by an arbitrary insurance company network list enforcer.

2. No network means no lists to consult when it comes to figuring out what providers to use, no risk of nasty surprises when seeking treatment away from home or in an emergency situation.

3. A patient covered by a Medicare supplement may seek treatment from any specialist anywhere without requesting permission from a gate-keeper or primary care physician.

4. Medicare supplement plans, just like Medicare Parts A & B, are good anywhere in the 50 US states and possessions. The plans I recommend also have a $50,000 lifetime benefit for emergency treatment in foreign countries.

5. Medicare supplements are guaranteed renewable and will provide their benefits forever, just as long as premiums continue to be paid. The onset of critical illness will not cause the coverage to be changed or terminated. The insurance company must live up to all of its obligations but the policy holder's only obligation is to continue payments when due.

6. A cautionary note: After your initial period of guaranteed issue eligibility, insurance companies may question your medical history if you apply for a different plan or to a different company. My advice is to choose your insurance carrier and your supplement plan very carefully because you just may have that plan for the rest of your life.

How does one decide which of the twelve Medicare supplement plans to purchase?

Follow my recommendation to buy either the luxurious Cadillac or the high-performance Pontiac of Medicare supplement plans.

LOTS OF BANG FOR REASONABLE BUCKS!

Two Medicare supplement plans I recommend for the average consumer:

The most comprehensive coverage allowed by law; the luxurious Cadillac of Medicare supplements:

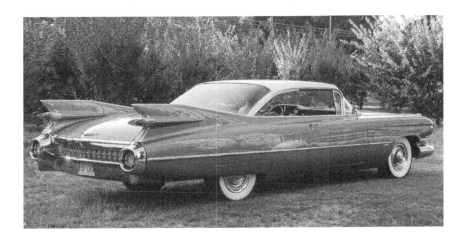

PLAN G for those born in 1955 or later

(**PLAN F** for those who are older, although probably not worth the extra premium cost)

-OR -

Great protection at an exceedingly low price: the high-performance Pontiac GTO of Medicare Supplements:

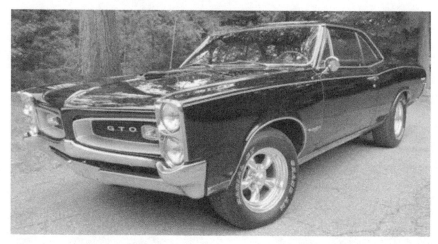

HIGH DEDUCTIBLE PLAN G if born in 1955 or later

(HIGH DEDUCTIBLE PLAN F for those who are older; it has identical benefits)

Each of these Medicare supplement plans covers 100% of the following costs (except the Part B deductible as noted), filling the many gaps in original Medicare:

Part A deductible

Part A coinsurance and hospital costs (to an additional 365 days after Medicare benefits are exhausted)

Part A hospice care coinsurance or copayment

Part B deductible – NOT covered by Plan G

Part B coinsurance or copayment

Part B excess charges

32

Skilled nursing facility coinsurance

Blood (first 3 pints)

AND:

80% of foreign travel emergency expenses after a small deductible (to a $50,000 lifetime total)

PLAN F has no deductibles, co-pays, co-insurance nor any other cost sharing provisions. The insured person will not receive any invoices for routine cost sharing expenses. You cannot buy this plan if you were born in 1955 or after.

PLAN G will reimburse everything but the Part B deductible ($226 in 2023).

Plans **HDF** and **HDG** credit the above expenses to their deductibles until they are met, and then pay at 100% for the rest of the year.

Here is more about <u>my favorite Medicare Supplement plans.</u> **High Deductible Plan F**, which those born before 1955 may continue to buy, but is priced higher than HDG by some companies.

Newest is High Deductible Plan G which is available to all who are Medicare eligible. These two supplement plans provide identical benefits.

LET'S CALL THEM "HIGH VALUE PLANS"

Both of the high deductible plans are saddled with an unfortunate and scary name. The insured will NOT have to pay the first $2,700 of medical expenses, only the much smaller Part A or Part B deductibles, depending on the type of medical treatment required.

After that, if the treatment continues, Medicare pays the vast majority of the expenses while the High Deductible plan applies the smaller unpaid segment of the expenses to its deductible, leaving the practitioners to send invoices for those relatively small amounts to the insured.

The insured typically has been saving as much as $100 per month by not buying an expensive Plan G (or F) so kicking in a few bucks here and there still leaves him with plenty of lettuce in his wallet.

Unless one is thrown into a hospital, these small invoices will be for 20% of the outpatient charges considered to be Medicare Part B expenses. Part B has an annual $226 deductible (in 2023) and then a 20% coinsurance for Part B treatment costs so individuals covered by the high deductible plans will pay 20% of their charges out-of-pocket in exchange for saving substantial premium dollars.

I illustrate in Chapter 9 that the term **"high deductible"** is a **complete misnomer,** since Medicare pays benefits no matter what supplement plan – if any – is in place.

This is why the term **"HIGH VALUE PLANS"** is much more accurate!

CHAPTER 9

The best kept secret in Medicare:
High Deductible "high value" plans!

High deductible plans are a terrific bargain! Too bad most agents won't talk about them. You see, they would rather earn hefty commissions than to give valuable advice that might cut into their earnings and save the client some money. The fact is, agents earn more when the product they sell is more costly!

The official description of these plans is that they have a hefty $2,700 "annual deductible" before picking up the balance of all unpaid medical bills. This completely ignores the fact that Medicare will begin paying the bills right after its very small deductible has been covered.

The insured WILL NOT PAY THE FIRST $2,700 (in 2023) of medical bills if they get sick or hurt! Medicare will pay the lion's share of the bills after the relatively small Part A/Part B deductibles (depending on the kind of treatment needed). The insured will pay a much smaller percentage of the bills until, in the unlikely event of a very bad year, his small portion adds up to the plan deductible. After that – 100% baby!

The name "high deductible" is completely misleading and the downside risk is so very limited that the average person will be flush with extra cash from the first month after buying the HD plan! The reality is that Medicare will have been paying 80% of outpatient expenses starting right after that $226 deductible!

This is why "HIGH VALUE" is a much better name!

Do you remember the beautiful days before Obamacare changed the health insurance landscape, driving up costs and removing many of the choices people could make? Most people had a medical plan that imposed a small deductible first, then a co-insurance or cost sharing period and finally began to pick up 100% of medical bills for the rest of the year.

For instance, a common plan could be described as having a $250 deductible, 80/20% co-insurance of the next $5000 and 100% thereafter. This was almost universal until this millenium and did a good job of protecting people from otherwise painful medical bills.

A smart Medicare Supplement purchaser may keep a similar level of protection, and at a very small monthly premium charge. A person buying the High Deductible Plans G (or F) will have something like a $226 deductible, then 80/20% of the next $12,000 and then 100% coverage for the rest of the year.

MEDICARE WILL ALWAYS PAY ITS PORTION FIRST.

Medicare doesn't know whether there is a supplement or not, it just goes along paying its 80% of the outpatient bills (after the $226 deductible).

For Part A expenses, it pays all of the first 2 months of hospital charges after the $1,600 (per admission) deductible. This means Medicare pays 100% of hospital costs after a reasonable deductible and 80% coverage for outpatient expenses after a small deductible, even if there is no supplement in place.

In the rare event of a disastrous series of medical events, the downside risk of High Deductible "high value" plans is very reasonable indeed.

As stated elsewhere, this book is written with a particular audience in mind: those who are not destitute and who are probably not infirm. This group can generally afford to pay the reasonable price of regular Plan G, the Cadillac and most popular of Medicare supplement plans. However, as comprehensive as the benefits of G are, they may not be the most cost-effective choice.

My healthy clients always appreciate the cost/benefit of High Deductible (or High Value) plans once it is properly explained to them that the term "high deductible" is a complete misnomer. When we are talking about outpatient Part B expenses, what we really have is a $226 deductible and 20% coinsurance of the next $12,370. After that the plan pays 100% for the rest of the year.

It is extremely unlikely that the average person will have total bills anywhere near $12,000. That means he will be saving somewhere near $100 per month year after year by choosing a High Deductible "High Value" plan. So, in a good year, the policy owner will likely save $1200 or more in comparison to the much higher cost of Plan G.

What if disaster strikes and medical expenses grow to a very large number in a given year? The insured person has plenty of downside protection from nasty surprises. If he has to spend all of that $2700 out of pocket towards the deductible and coinsurance, remember that he very likely saved $1200 in premium costs so that leaves just over $1200 (or about $100 per month on the average) to meet his share until the High Deductible plan starts paying 100% for the rest of the year.

What about the monthly savings the insured enjoyed for the many years that expensive medical treatment was not needed? ...and what about the many years of good health and monthly savings that will follow that one unfortunate year?

MONEY IN THE BANK!

CHAPTER 10

Medicare Advantage (Part C) Plans: Why Not?

The only advantage I can see in Medicare Advantage plans is that they don't cost very much to buy. In fact, many of them have $0 monthly premiums! Good deal, right?

Sure, they can be a pretty good deal if nothing bad happens to you; no serious injury or illness that causes the need for medical treatment. In other words, you will be just fine with a Medicare Advantage plan until you actually need to use it. Then you may discover why some people refer to them as "Medicare Dis-advantage plans".

Insurance agents love these plans because of the generous commissions they pay (thanks to the largess of the taxpayers). Why should you, the insurance buyer beware the hidden booby-traps in Medicare Advantage plans? Where are the flaws in Medicare Advantage or Part C plans for the potential customers like you?

The big one: NO FREEDOM OF CHOICE!

1. MEDICARE ADVANTAGE (Part C) plans are HMOs or PPOs. They all rely on networks of physicians and hospitals to deliver care. This adds the complication of having to choose your provider from their list of names to ensure treatment will be covered.

2. One is encouraged do comparison shopping every year because important elements of MA plans are constantly in flux, with some changes occurring mid-year. If your favorite doctor were to quit your network, you would be stuck finding a replacement from the list given to you by the insurance company. Plans that include drug coverage will often change their formularies, sometimes rendering the

whole plan a great deal more expensive.

3. The average Advantage plan has an out-of-pocket limit of $8300 per year with some having a limit as high as $11,300 for in-network expenses. If the plan has any coverage for out-of-network expenses, the maximum out-of-pocket this year is $12,450. Why would anyone be uncomfortable with a Medicare Supplement High Deductible (High Value) plan out-of-pocket limit of $2700 by comparison to that much higher possible loss?

4. Even the most highly touted Advantage plans can beat an insured to death with hidden fees and co-pays. One best-selling plan in Florida has co-pays like this: ambulance: $300; hospital stay: $175 per day for first 10 days; diabetic supplies: 20% coinsurance; diagnostic radiology: up to $125 co-pay; lab services: $100 per day; outpatient X-rays: up to $100 per day; therapeutic radiology: $35 up to 20% co-pay; renal dialysis: 20% of the actual fee.

5. Costly complications can spring out of the bushes to cause unpleasant surprises. For example, your surgeon might belong to the network but the anesthesiologist he uses may not; the radiologist may be in the network but the specialists who interpret the films may not be. In these examples, you should expect to receive a hefty invoice in the mail. This problem was addressed by federal legislation in 2022 but I have been told that implementation of the new protections is very slow.

6. Frequently, permission is required prior to seeking consultation with a specialist. This permission is often provided by a primary care physician (PCP) who insists on a scheduled appointment before providing that permission.

   A lengthy investigation by the Inspector General of the Department of HHS recently caught a number of these plans denying requests of this nature to all subscribers and then rolling over to change that decision for the small minority who displayed the moxie to file grievances. The other suffering members? I guess they either went without treatment or paid out-of-pocket.

7. Networks usually operate in a localized area and traveling out of it or living in a second home somewhere can be a problem, if medical treatment is needed.

8. They will promise that out-of-network emergency care is covered, but may balk at cooperating when it comes to paying for it.

9. Insurance agents who try to enroll hapless victims into a "low cost" or "free" Advantage plan will then sometimes badger them to purchase additional Hospital Indemnity insurance to pay the hidden expenses not covered by the Advantage plan.

10. The many extras they tout, like dental, vision and hearing coverage are often disappointing limited benefit discount plans rather than true insurance coverage. In addition, they rely on small networks of doctors and dentists, further restricting freedom of choice.

SOMETIMES WE GET WHAT WE PAY FOR!

How can an insurance company give away a product for free? This only works if the government pays the freight. When the government decides to cut its expenses, the insured clients will be the ones to pick up the slack. In the meantime, very large commissions mean that you will never cease hearing about the wonderful world of Medicare Advantage from insurance agents.

The good news is that holders of Medicare Advantage (Part C) plans are allowed to switch from one plan or company to another every year during AEP or Open Enrollment, which allows dissatisfied subscribers to try out a new plan to be effective the following January 1st.

Have you noticed that there is a huge amount of direct mail, TV ads, internet pop-ups and other annoying insurance talk happening every fall? This is because the poor saps who found themselves stuck with Medicare Advantage plans have an opportunity to try a different MA plan.... anything else to replace the crapola they bought last year.

Once again, **I do not recommend these plans** for my audience of Medicare eligibles who are not destitute or infirm.

CHAPTER 11

MEDICARE MSA:

An Advantage plan I actually like!

Freedom of choice is rare in the Medicare Advantage world, but I have found an MA plan that might just cure that problem!

The standard MA (Part C) plans that flood your mailbox and assault your eyeballs often advertise themselves to be free of charge or have $0 premium. How do you think an insurance plan is able to assume the risk that an older person will need expensive medical treatment without charging a premium each month?

The answer? They receive cash directly from the government.

They use this money to pay medical providers, provide cheapo dental and vision coverage plus pretend to offer a bunch of other stuff to get people interested in signing up for eventual disappointment.

How do we know there is likely to be disappointment? Just look at the frenzied level of activity every October to December when all of these poor saps have an opportunity to dump their plan and try a different one.

Turns out 53 days in each fall wasn't long enough to satisfy the demand for freedom so the period has been extended into the new year, probably to avoid the risk of armed insurrection.

I have seen a glimmer of light on the horizon! It just might prove to be salvation for the Medicare Advantage industry.

It is a very dim light so far, but hope springs eternal!

This unusual product is a **Medicare MSA or "Medical Savings Account"** and it offers some of the best of both worlds: Advantage and Supplement in such a way that I can almost bring myself to recommend it.

The only thing stopping me from enthusiastic endorsement is the caution one feels after having seen so many high hopes dashed over the years.

The one Medicare MSA company with which I am most familiar is indeed offering a Medicare Advantage plan in the sense that its funds come from the government.

However, instead of keeping all that money while offering worthless baubles and empty promises to potential subscribers, this MSA actually gives a chunk of the funding directly to the subscriber. By "chunk" I mean thousands and thousands of US greenbacks.

This is the way one MSA plan works:

Medicare (the US government) gives the plan an infusion of funds; the plan then deposits some cash into a bank account in your name. It uses some of the rest to purchase a high deductible health insurance policy that pays 100% after the deductible. The balance of their funds is used for agent's commission, operating revenue and profit.

Here is what you, the purchaser of the plan will see:

1. A $0 premium health insurance plan with no restrictive network of doctors and hospitals. Any provider that accepts Medicare payment can be consulted anytime the patient chooses.

2. An annual deposit of either $2,000 or $3,000 (your choice) into a bank account in your name. How you spend, save or invest this money is entirely up to you.

3. A high deductible insurance policy will provide a ceiling on the amount at risk in the event of catastrophic medical expenses. The deductible will either be $5,000 or $8,000 for the year, depending on the amount of annual deposit for which you signed up.

4. The opportunity to roll over that deposit to the following year when another deposit will be made to your account, or withdraw the remaining funds in the account, pay income taxes and splurge on the rest.

5. The need to purchase the Prescription Drug Plan of your choice. If you have no regular prescription meds, a Part D drug plan in your area will be very inexpensive. Since this is based on your residence location, I will be able to identify the cheapest plan in your area upon request.

My understanding is that several companies offer Medicare MSAs in their local regions. I only know of one company that operates in a multi-state, almost nationwide environment.

Until there is a demonstrated level of performance and stability, I am reluctant to broadly endorse the concept or the only Medicare MSA carrier I am contracted with.

If you want to take a closer look at this health insurance plan with a savings account component and an element of risk, contact me at my podcast e-mail address and I will send you a brochure: DBJ@MLMMailbag.com.

Freedom is a great thing; cross your fingers that it spreads across the land and defeats the evil Advantage monster!

CHAPTER 12

Drugs? We Don't Need No Stinkin' Drugs!

PDP, Prescription Drug Plan or Part D

– buy it ASAP!

In their infinite generosity, the Feds now subsidize the cost of prescription drug plans that can be purchased from private insurance companies. Each of these companies can price their drug plans where they want to, compile their own list of drugs to be covered (formularies) and offer different levels of benefit to their customers.

Here are the problems: the construction of each drug plan sounds very complicated to the non-insurance professional; there are deductibles, co-pays, co-insurance and a big scary donut hole to contend with.

Additionally, the formularies and premiums can change from one year to the next and each individual's prescription medication requirements can change.

Therefore, I recommend comparing all available plans only on the basis of the estimated total out of pocket cost per year. If the changes in formulary, premium cost or drug needs warrant, the insured can select a new plan from another company during the annual open enrollment period for the following year.

There is a fairly painless way to compare the cost of all of the drug plans in your locality via the government website. Look for the easy navigation directions below.

What if you are so healthy that you take no prescription drugs at all? After thanking the ancestors who passed down your particular gene pool, consider whether there might be a need for insuring against high prescription costs anytime in the future. If not, and you expect to never, ever purchase one of these drug plans, you are finished right now.

On the other hand, most people without crystal balls like to keep their options open and hedge their bets. And they generally want to avoid the lifetime late enrollment penalty.

If a person becomes eligible to purchase a PDP but elects not to do that, and then decides to go ahead and buy one sometime in the future, a late enrollment penalty will be assessed for each month elapsed from the initial eligibility period to the actual purchase.

The penalty amounts to roughly 35 cents per month for each month elapsed. That means an extra $4.20 per month for a one-year delay, $8.40 per month for a two-year delay, $12.60 per month for a three-year delay and so on.

This is why I advise my clients to buy an inexpensive PDP when they are first eligible, even if they take no drugs yet. A price war makes it difficult for me to guess the likely price but if you contact me with your residence address I will identify the cheapest in your county.

Admittedly, not all have followed my advice, but I sleep better at night knowing that I tried.

Kind of like child rearing.

EASY DIY NAVIGATION INSTRUCTIONS TO SELECT THE LOWEST COST PDP:

Go to site: https://www.medicare.gov/plan-compare

1) In lower right quadrant, click: **Select Plan Type**
   Choose: **Drug Plan (Part D)**

   Click: **Apply**

2) Enter residence **ZIP Code** – Choose your county if necessary.

3) Click: **START**

4) Next question (on left side): Do you get help with your costs from one of these programs?
   What follows is a list of six options – Select the last item:
   I don't get help from any of these programs.

5) Click: **Next**

6) Tell us your search preferences; Do you want to see your drug costs when you compare plans?

   A: **Yes** (Start with "A" Below)

   B: **No:** No drugs taken. (Skip to "B" below)

7) Click: **Next**

A) Begin typing in box to find and select your drug;
Follow prompts to select dosage, quantity, frequency

Click: **Add to My Drug List**; repeat for other drugs

Click: **Done adding drugs**

Chose up to five pharmacies; type names in box and/or
search below

Click: **check box next to each pharmacy**

Click: **"Done" to the right of pharmacy list**

Click: **"Add to Compare"** box on first three plans

Click: **"Compare"** to the right

Final screen shows three plans with lowest total cost for
balance of calendar year

Ask Doug for guidance enrolling: DBJ@MLMMailbag.com

B) Click: **No (No drugs taken)**

Click: **Next**

On the following screen, scroll down to the first plan:

that is the cheapest prescription drug plan for the rest of the
year.

Ask Doug for guidance enrolling: DBJ@MLMMailbag.com

If you were successful in following these directions you will have identified the least costly Part D prescription drug plan available in your county. The measurement is the plan with the lowest out-of-pocket cost. This cost is a combination of the plan premium PLUS the co-pays charged on your drugs when prescriptions are filled at your preferred pharmacies and/or the plan's mail-order service. Do not let a very high or very low plan premium influence your decision unduly.

Once you have selected the plan (or plans) you want to consider, you may click: Details in order to learn more, but remember that the prime goal here is to select the plan with the lowest out-of-pocket cost at the pharmacies you wish to patronize. If you wish to self-enroll, call the "non-members" number to accomplish that.

On the other hand, if you want to throw a few shekels into the retirement fund of yours truly, send an e-mail to me: DBJ@MLMMailbag.com and if contracted with your chosen plan, I will handle your enrollment.

Consider repeating this process next year at the Annual Enrollment Period (AEP) in the fall to ensure you have the lowest cost plan.

CHAPTER 13

What Will All of This Cost?

There is a monetary cost for all insurance coverage and government supplied health insurance is no exception. The good news is that, if you are coming off an Obamacare type of plan, the new costs will look like a bargain to you!

A note about IRMAA – the success penalty. This stands for Income Related Monthly Adjustment Amount and may add to the monthly premium for Medicare Part B and for the Prescription Drug Plan, based on what the IRS has recorded as your MAGI (Modified Adjusted Gross Income) two years ago.

The target audience for this book is likely to encounter the following monthly premium costs in 2023:

Medicare Part A

Free of Charge (after 40 quarters of taxable earnings)

Medicare Part B

$164.90 (IRMAA could increase it substantially)

Medicare Supplement Plans: Premiums vary widely depending on several factors. These include state of residence, age, sex, ZIP Code and sometimes smoking status, height & weight.

HIGH DEDUCTIBLE (high value) PLANS F or G -

Most cost effective – estimated between $30 and $80

PLAN F –

Most comprehensive -estimated between $160 & $300

PLAN G -

Much lower priced than Plan F but Part B deductible ($226) is not covered

PDP –

Prescription Drug Plans - $1.50 and up, depending on plan and location plus drug deductibles, co-pay and co-insurance.

PDP premiums are also subject to an IRMAA penalty assessment.

2023 MEDICARE COST SHARING PROVISIONS

PART A - Deductible and co-insurance payable by you or your Supplement

Deductible per hospital admission = You pay $1,600
Co-insurance hospital days 1 to 60 = You pay $0
Co-insurance days 61 to 90 = You pay $400 per day Co-insurance days 91 to 150 = You pay $800 per day_
Skilled Nursing Facility:
Co-insurance days 0 to 20 = You pay $0
Co-insurance days 21 to 100 = You pay $200/day

PART B – Deductible and co-insurance payable by you or your Supplement

Annual Deductible = $226
Co-insurance (no limit) = 20%

IRMAA

2023 IRMAA PENALTIES – Part B and Part D

Based on MAGI (Modified Adjusted Gross Income) 2 years prior

Single	Married Filing Jointly	Married Filing Separately	Part B IRMAA PREMIUM	Part D IRMAA PENALTY
$97,000 or less	$194,000 or less	$97,000 or less	$164.90	$0 + your plan premium
$97,000 to $123,000	$194,000 to $246,000	N/A	$230.80	$12.20 + your plan premium
$123,000 to $153,000	$246,000 to $306,000	N/A	$329.70	$31.50 + your plan premium
$153,000 to $183,000	$306,000 to $366,000	N/A	$428.60	$50.70 + your plan premium
$183,000 and under $500,000	$366,000 and under $750,000	$97,000 and under $403,000	$527.50	$70.00 + your plan premium
$500,000 or above	$750,000 and above	$403,000 and above	$560.60	$76.40 + your plan premium

CHAPTER 14

MASSACHUSETTS, MINNESOTA & WISCONSIN

The three states addressed here somehow managed to persuade the Federal Government to grant waivers allowing them to create their own Medicare Supplement plans. All of the general characteristics that make supplements superior to Advantage plans still apply to these outliers. For example, they work anywhere in the United States and they have no restrictive doctor or hospital networks.

Otherwise, the benefit structure of these state designed plans differs markedly from the Medicare Supplement plans we have discussed that are available in the other 47. The following descriptions are drawn, in part, from www.medicare.gov. To peruse the actual coverage details, go to that site and search "Medigap-in-(state)".

MASSACHUSETTS

The Bay State has three plans available. One may buy the Core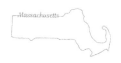

Plan or either Supplement 1 (only for

those born before 1955) or Supplement 1A. Each of them includes the same set of Basic Benefits.

Each supplement has additional elements that fill the gaps in Original Medicare plus some state mandated benefits. The bottom line is that the Core Plan is lean and probably much less costly as a stand-alone rather than buying a supplement.

Want to save money? Obviously, the Core Plan is going to be less expensive than a Supplement Plan, no matter which insurance company is offering them. The only strategy I can see is to carefully examine the additional benefits covered by the Supplement 1 or 1A Plans to decide for yourself if the savings in premium dollars by purchasing only the Core Plan would be worth the risk.

As an example, you may not plan to travel abroad, or you have no expectation of being committed to a mental hospital. These are coverages you likely can avoid paying for without concern. However, you would want to think carefully about savings vs. risk of going without coverage for the Part A hospital deductible or the skilled nursing facility coinsurance.

Compare these plans side-by-side

If a "yes" appears, the plan covers the described benefit 100%. If "no" appears, the policy doesn't cover that benefit.

Medigap Benefits	Medigap Plans		
	Core Plan	Supplement 1	Supplement 1A
Basic benefits	Yes	Yes	Yes
Part A: inpatient hospital deductible	No	Yes	Yes
Part A: skilled nursing facility coinsurance	No	Yes	Yes
Part B: deductible*	No	Yes*	No
Foreign travel emergency	No	Yes	Yes
Inpatient days in mental health hospitals	60 days per calendar year	120 days per benefit year	120 days per benefit year
State-mandated benefits (yearly Pap tests and mammograms. Check your plan for other state-mandated benefits.)	No	Yes	Yes

MINNESOTA

In the North Star State there is a plethora of Medicare Supplement plans available for sale.

The Basic and Extended Basic plans are described in the chart below. They are available when you enroll in Part B, regardless of your age or health problems.

Compare these plans side-by-side

If a "yes" appears, the plan covers the described benefit 100%. If a row lists a percentage, the policy covers that percentage of the described benefit. If a "no" appears, the policy doesn't cover that benefit.

Medigap Benefits	Medigap Plans	
	Basic Plan	Extended Basic Plan
Basic benefits	Yes	Yes
Part A: inpatient hospital deductible	No	Yes
Part A: skilled nursing facility coinsurance	Yes (Provides 100 days of SNF care)	Yes (Provides 120 days of SNF care)
Part B: deductible**	No	Yes**
Foreign travel emergency	80%	80%*
Outpatient mental health	50%	50%
Usual and customary fees	No	80%*
Medicare-cover preventative care	Yes	Yes
Physical therapy	20%	20%
Coverage while in a foreign country	No	80%*
State-mandated benefits (diabetic equipment and supplies, routine cancer screening, reconstructive surgery, and immunizations)	Yes	Yes

Insurance companies may offer 4 additional riders that can be added to a Basic Plan. You may choose any or all of these riders to design a policy that meets your needs:

1. Part A deductible

2. Part B deductible (only for those eligible for Medicare but not enrolled before 2020)

3. Usual and customary fees

4. Non-Medicare preventive care

Minnesota versions of Medicare Supplement plans K, L, M, N plus a High Deductible Plan are also available.

I would take a close look at High Deductible Plan as these usually offer the most cost-effective Medicare protection..

WISCONSIN

The Badger State has taken a build-your-own approach to Medicare Supplement coverage.

Of course, there are the ever-present Basic Benefits but they are included in the Basic Plan which also covers:

1. Part A: skilled nursing facility coinsurance

2. 175 days per lifetime in addition to Medicare's benefit of inpatient mental health coverage

3. 40 additional home health care visits

4. State mandated benefits

Insurance companies are also allowed to offer these riders:

- Part A deductible

- 365 additional home health care visits

- Part B deductible

- Part B excess charges

- Foreign travel emergency

- 50% Part A deductible

- Part B copayment or coinsurance

There is also a High Deductible, high value plan available.

If I were shopping for a Medicare Supplement in Wisconsin, that high value plan would be the first thing I would look at.

CHAPTER 15

The only chapter you are likely to need!

Are you in charge of your own health insurance and hoping to simplify the Medicare coverage selection process?

The next few pages will allow you to ignore the prevailing confusion and purchase the best, most comprehensive medical insurance available.

STEP 1.

Have you selected your Medicare Part A start date?
(Read more in Chapter 4)

Have you selected your Medicare Part B start date?
(Read more in Chapter 5)

ENROLL IN MEDICARE ONLINE HERE:
https://www.ssa.gov/medicare/
Scroll down to find the blue button that says:

Apply for Medicare Only

The enrollment process could take as little as 10 minutes.

Only two more steps to go!

STEP 2.

Decide on and apply for your Medicare supplement plan.

For this step you need a licensed insurance agent. If you would like me to act as your agent, send an email:

DBJ@MLMMailbag.com

I will then send you a very short questionnaire in order to learn enough to prepare accurate quotes.

If you prefer, go to my website and scroll down to the orange

"Get a Quote" or "Apply Now" buttons.

Information you provide here will be sent immediately to me in complete security.

www.MedicareForTheLazyMan.com

What follows are descriptions of the two types of Medicare supplement plans I recommend and sell:

CHOOSE YOUR MEDICARE SUPPLEMENT PLAN

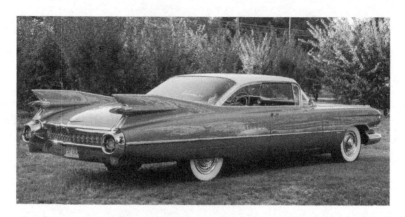

LUXURIOUS CADILLAC OF MEDICARE SUPPLEMENT PLANS

Most comprehensive coverage. Best suited for those with comfortable finances, low risk tolerance and desiring 100% coverage no matter the cost.

PLAN F: Formerly the most popular choice and only available to those born before 1955. This has the highest monthly premium and the richest benefit structure. PLAN F pays 100% of all deductibles, co-pays and co-insurance. The insured will not receive any invoices for cost sharing expenses when all medical treatment is Medicare approved.

Unfortunately, my observation is that insurance companies are raising the rates on Plan F drastically.

PLAN G: Set to become the most popular choice and certainly the richest benefit structure after PLAN F. Pays all of the expenses listed above except for the annual $226 Part B annual deductible. This is the simplest and richest plan available to those first becoming eligible for Medicare in 2020 or later.

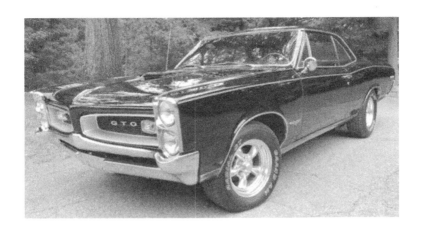

HIGH PERFORMANCE PONTIAC GTO OF MEDICARE SUPPLEMENT PLANS
– most cost-effective coverage

Best suited for those having somewhat higher risk tolerance, willing to accept some limited cost sharing expenses in return for a substantially lower monthly premium cost.

HIGH DEDUCTIBLE PLANS G & F:

Cover all of the risks of legitimate expenses as are covered by PLANS G & F above. However, instead of paying at 100% from day one of each year, they pay at something less than 100% with the insured making up the relatively small difference.

In the unlikely event of very high medical expenses, the plan starts paying 100% after the insured's portion adds up to $2,700 (in 2023).

 Substantially lower monthly premium than Plans G or F.

READ MORE ABOUT MEDICARE SUPPLEMENT PLANS IN CHAPTERS 7, 8 & 9

STEP 3.
Select the least expensive Prescription Drug Plan (PDP) from a list of all plans available in your area.

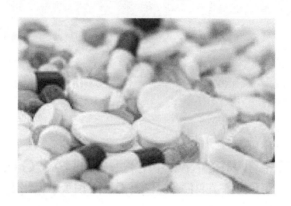

Purchase that plan online directly from the insurance company.

In Chapter 12 you will find step-by-step DIY navigation instructions leading you to that list of PDP plans arranged in order of annual cost.

These instructions look complicated, but it is a government website and so was not designed to be user-friendly. The most complicated part of the process will be entering the detail for each of your current prescription medications.

Since the PDPs are one-year contracts, annual costs can change at the discretion of each insurance company. Also, your prescription drug needs may change during the course of the year.

Therefore, you may find this a worthwhile project to do each year during the Annual Election Period (AEP) in the fall, in case you would like to buy a new plan for the following year.

EASY NAVIGATION INSTRUCTIONS TO SELECT AND PURCHASE A LOW-COST PDP:

THE STEPS ARE ILLUSTRATED IN CHAPTER 12!

If you were successful, CONGRATULATIONS! Your Medicare prescription drug plan (PDP) work is done!

Furthermore, if you were able to complete all three of these steps, you now have acquired the four essential elements of protection:

MEDICARE PART A

    MEDICARE PART B

        MEDICARE SUPPLEMENT PLANS

            PRESCRIPTION DRUG PLANS

CHAPTER 16

Did You Make a Boo-Boo?

It is very possible that you are hearing about the excellent benefits of Medicare supplement plans and especially the great cost advantage of High Deductible "High Value" PLANS for the first time.

Since commissions payable to agents are more substantial for Medicare Advantage plans, those are the ones that are promoted most vigorously to the unsuspecting public.

Is that the case with you?

Were you kept in the dark about Medicare supplements and High Deductible, "High Value" plans?

Are you anxious to make a change so that you can enjoy the benefits of Medicare supplement plans along with all of my happy clients?

Well, I have good news and bad news for you:

GOOD NEWS: You may apply for a Medicare supplement policy from an insurance carrier any time the mood strikes!

BAD NEWS: There is no "guaranteed issue" period for Medicare supplement plans after your initial enrollment period when you first became eligible. You MAY be asked a series of questions about your medical history in order to prove that you are insurable.

This is not true in every instance or in every state but generally you will have to jump through some hoops in order to be allowed to buy a Medicare supplement policy outside of the initial enrollment period. You might be refused if your medical condition and history do not meet the insurance company's insurability standards.

There are a few special exceptions but understanding them and the related complexities is what makes Medicare so much fun.

I may be able to help, and I would like to try!

CONTACT ME:

DBJ@MLMmailbag.com

www.MedicareForTheLazyMan.com

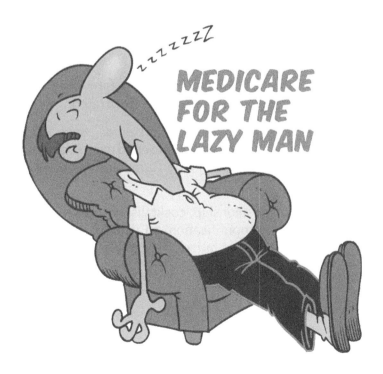

ACKNOWLEDGMENTS

This book would not exist. I would still be sitting at my desk with fingers poised over the keys and eyes caressing the mountains around our Arizona home were it not for my wife.

Mary is among my most rabid critics but can often be brought around to my way of thinking with some persistent persuasion. Once on my team, she is an invaluable asset and a source of insight, inspiration, motivation and support.

Mary is not really high maintenance, but she does need to be reminded periodically that "spousal unit" is actually a term of loving endearment. Not much else to say after almost 50 years of partnership and teamwork.

Thanks to my personal clients who helped me form the idea for this project after realizing why they were all so frustrated.

Others, generally without being pestered, have explained complicated technological mysteries, prodded me out of lethargy or sharpened red pencils to gleefully perform surgery on my sterling prose.

They have shared companionship, cocktails, encouragement, ribald jokes and philosophical pontification, all without ever a negative word about this relatively ambitious project. So I also thank, in no particular order:

Randy & Margaret Carson of C2C Consulting, LLC
Brian and Teri Jones
Gerry and Lisa Schafer
Paul and Kathleen Bowling
Tony and Melisa Coletto
Roy & Kathy Brotherhood

Finally, for no reason other than I just enjoy them, I must acknowledge the youngest generation of my gene pool. Thanks for making the rest of us proud and happy to have you in our family:

Max Coletto & Alex Coletto Californians just starting to spread their wings.
Drew, Magda and baby Nora McMillin
Robbie McMillin and Kate McMillin –
Canadian-Americans proud to wave both flags!

ABOUT THE AUTHOR

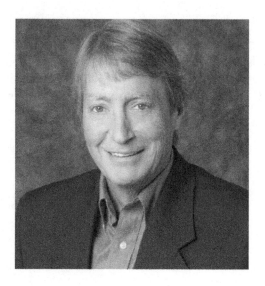

Douglas B. Jones, CLU, RHU

Medicare snuck up on me just as it does with most Americans.

As a long-time health insurance professional, I was expected by friends and clients to be ahead of the curve. Turns out I needed to educate myself on this complex subject in order to be able to offer solid advice.

After graduation from the University of Arizona I joined my family's John Hancock insurance agency in Chicago's Loop. Even though life insurance sales with the John Hancock was a 3-generation family calling, I found more satisfaction in helping clients with their health insurance needs.

Eventually the company stopped offering those products so I left to pursue my mission with other companies.

Decades later at a social event, I was asked by several people for a short version of my Medicare advice. They assumed I must be an expert since we were all rapidly approaching age 65.

That was the catalyst that convinced me to learn what Medicare was all about. After a period of study, I formed some conclusions that are directly at odds with other Medicare advisors.

One evening a couple of longtime friends came over to act as my Guinea pigs. The wife, ever the serious student, was lugging all of the printed material they had received and expected me to educate them on every one of the Medicare options available in our area.

The husband was mostly interested in the beer I offered. His opinion was that this whole Medicare decision process was an unpleasant inconvenience that should end quickly.

Very soon, these friends had a complete grasp of my best Medicare advice and the reasons behind it. They were stunned that the whole thing could be boiled down to such a simple conclusion. As they discovered, the most time-consuming part of the process was completing the insurance paperwork.

That evening set the pattern for virtually all of my subsequent encounters with Medicare eligible citizens. Years later it occurred to me that the same process could be offered to everyone in the country who was staring down the barrel of Medicare.

Thus, was born *Medicare for the Lazy Man*!

Made in United States
Orlando, FL
28 July 2023

35545298R00046